"Native American Medicine: A guide to natural healing for your body"

TABLE OF CONTENT

I0419827

INTRODUCTION

For thousands of years, man has made use of alternative medicine to cure illnesses, fight viruses and find solutions to stubborn diseases. For thousands of years, these methods have been carefully developed, researched and preserved, so it can be useful for generations to come. Then came modern civilization and its many complexes and guiding principles, about the right standards for human existence, and everything changed.

Native American medicine used to be a very important part of human existence in Northern America. It was a solid vital component for the people as it ensures their healthy living and ability to fight off infections. Then came modern medicine and people will soon forget about the good things that has existed and was effective long ago. The will to make huge profits from people's illness has now become the major reasons for finding a solution to serious health problems.

In recent years, people are beginning to ask questions about what humans can benefit from the lifestyle of people who existed thousands of years ago. Based on research, these peoples have fewer medical problems compared with what we have today, and were able to manage good health with very little resources. Did these Native American people know what we do not know now? What is it that we can learn from them? Do they have the answers to some of the most dangerous health problems that we have today; including cancer, Ebola and HIV/AIDS?

One thing is certain, orthodox medicine has very serious limitations. If not, governments will not be spending billions ever year trying to stop diseases from eliminating the human population. If not, many people will not be on the sick bed with little or no hope for their ailment.

Our intention is to make you understand why it is important to seek for alternative medicine for your ailments. You will learn how to look for and find the perfect Native American medicine, how to work with skilled professionals and the benefits you will derive from using medicine that is in line with nature. You will also learn how using native medicine can help reduce the cost of your medical expenses.

CHAPTER 1

WHAT IS NATIVE AMERICAN MEDICINE?

Native American medicine is one of the many alternatives or traditional medicines that have been providing solutions to people's health issues for so many years ago. It majorly consists of the use of herbs and roots, but certain practices might also include cleansing of the spirit, soul and mind. Native American medicine is not as popular as other types of traditional medicine like Chinese, Korean and Indian native medicine because of its neglect by mainstream America. In recent years, people are beginning to pay attention to this wonderful alternative, which can provide solutions to some of the most dreaded illnesses we have in the world today.

A short history of Native American medicine

Thousands of years ago, Native Americans live very happily on the North American continents. There are approximately 2,000 tribes living side by side, with very similar traditional practices. To the natives, good health, just like now, is believed to be an important aspect of human life. This is why medicine men and women are highly respected and regarded as part of the tribes.

Native medicine practitioners make use of herbs, roots and rituals to heal people who are suffering from a wide range of illnesses. According to historical records, the healing methods were very effective. This is mainly because of its approach, which involves connecting the human spirit and at the same time applying physical herbs to cure the body. Native American medicines was far more advanced than the medicines of the European settlers; as many illnesses considered that are considered fatal, are easily cured by the natives.

Native American medicines are still very potent, although may not be as effective as it were, thousands of years ago. This is because practices differ throughout the 2,000 tribes, and passing down information was mainly committed to memory. In modern times, practitioners of the native medicine have truly modernized it, without sacrificing quality and potency.

Is native medicine for you?

Before venturing into native medicine, it is important that you consider your ailment first before any other thing. Have you tried other orthodox options and they did not work? Do you think that native medicine will help you save money? Are you just looking for an alternative medical solution with rich experiences that will connect your soul and body, and not just mere consumption of pills?

In addition to these questions, you will also need to consult a certified medical professional before you take any steps. This is to ensure that you are not self-medicating, which can be dangerous to your health. You should know that herbs react with each other and with other medicines in diverse ways. Your doctor will also be able to determine if you will be able to use your native medicine along with your prescription, to hasten your healing. You will also be able to get a detailed analysis of what you should be expecting as a patient at the end of the day.

CHAPTER 2

TYPES OF NATIVE AMERICAN MEDICINE AND THEIR USES

There are many Native American medicines, herbs and plants. This complexity makes it a little bit difficult for people looking for healing to focus their attention on a particular area. We have concluded on this list after examining some of the regularly used herbs, which have been tested and trusted by generation of users. Some of these herbs are also a part of medicines manufactured by pharmaceuticals.

The most effective of these is through the traditional preparation process that ensures that the energy inside the plants and herbs remain intact. Because if they don't, they may not work as you'd expect.

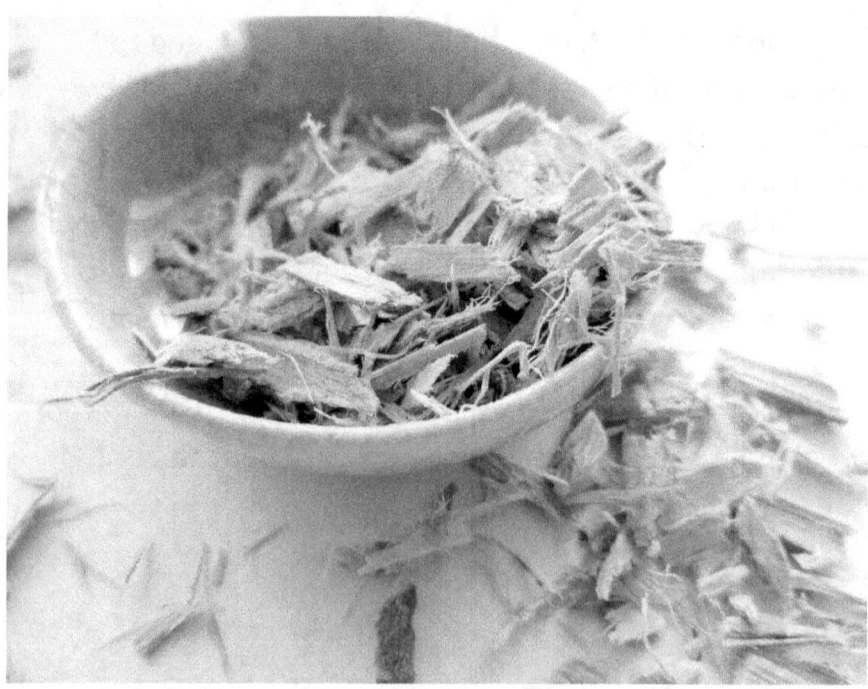

WILLOW BARK

Willow bark or basket willow or black willow extract is derived from the bark of willow trees, which is then made into medicine. In the past, the Native Americans chewed it, in order to get relief from pain, especially during healing. Willow bark contains an active ingredient known as Salicin. This is what gives it its aspirin-like effect, which makes it very effective for curing severe headaches, gout, muscle pain, rheumatic arthritis and menstrual cramp.

Willow bark is also very effective for the treatment of lower back pain, if taken in higher dosage. Research shows that people who take it for lower back pain and joint pain usually get relief after about a week or so. There are also unconfirmed evidence that it can help obese people lose weight when taken with kola nut.

How to use willow bark

There are two most reliable ways to take willow bark - supplements and tea. Supplements are good because they have been carefully prepared to match the exact amount of Salicin that should be in your body at a particular time. Willow bark tea is also very helpful, as it gives you the chance to consume the medicine at a very reasonable rate. You should note that it is not advisable to consume willow bark in its raw form or powdered form because of the effects of overdose.

Side effects of willow bark

Willow bark is a very useful medicine, but there are certain groups of people that should avoid it. For example, people who are suffering from diabetes should not use willow bark. If you are suffering from any diseases that does not allow you to use aspirin, you should also not use willow bark. People suffering from asthma, liver conditions, kidney problems peptic ulcer should not to use it. Women who are breastfeeding or pregnant are also advised not to use willow bark. Sometimes people want to use willow bark for children with flu or cold. It is advisable that you should not use it for children at all to avoid exposing them to Reye's syndrome. Willow's bark might lead to extra bleeding during and after surgery. Make sure that you stop taking it two weeks before going to surgery.

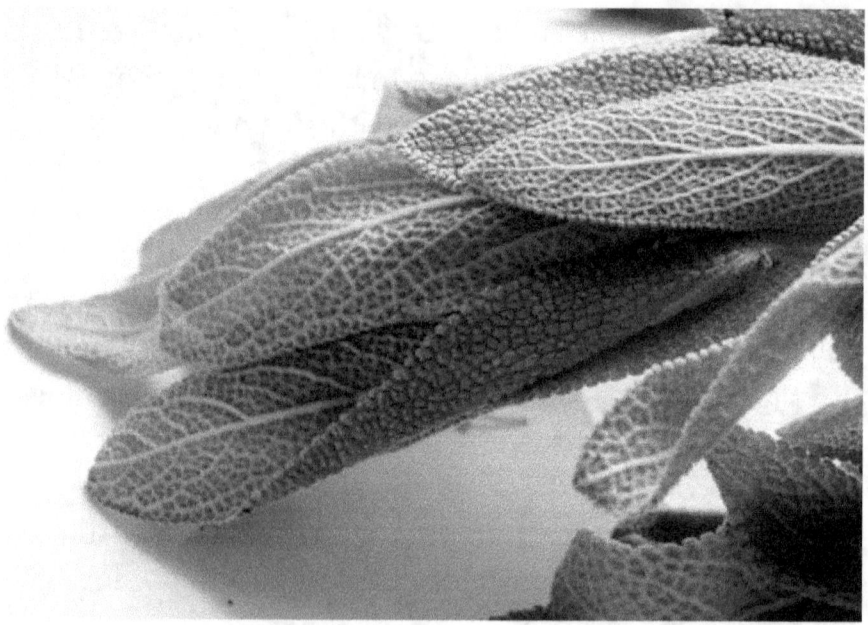

SAGE

Sage is one of the most useful Native American medicines, as its leaves are for medicine. It is for people suffering from digestive system complication, as it provides solutions for heartburn, flatulence, diarrhea, gastritis and bloating. It also helps in the treatment of Alzheimer's disease and loss of appetite.

Sage for Menstrual periods

Women who experience painful menstruation can use sage to get relief. It can also be very useful in the reducing hot flush during menopause. You can also use it to reduce excessive flow of milk in nursing mothers. It can also be very effective in the treatment of menopausal sweats.

Skin application

You can use Sage directly on the skin to help cure sores on the mouth, throat and tongue. You can also use it for gum disease, as well as painful and swollen nasal passages.

Treating wounds

Sometimes wounds are difficult to heal. The Native Americans lived an active life that included hunting and wars, so they were most likely going to get wounds very often. Sage, when applied to wounds, can facilitate the healing process and prevent the exposure to infections.

Other uses

Some asthmatic people also inhale sage to help reduce their symptoms. Sage contain ingredients that can help restructure chemical imbalances in the brain. This is why it is widely used in the treatment of Alzheimer's. For example, taking certain species of sage for a period of four months has improved the brain processing ability of people with mild cases of Alzheimer's.

Usage

Raw consumption and tea form is the most popular ways for taking sage. The sage tea guarantees quick assimilation of healing properties, while people who want to have a total feel of the herb's wonders can it eat raw. Sometimes, people make sage extracts. That is however not very common in practice.

Precautions for sage use

If you have diabetes and you're using sage, make sure that you monitor your blood sugar. This is because sage can lower blood sugar in diabetic people leading to low energy situations. Please note that a certain sage species known as Salvia Officinalis can trigger seizures. So, if you suffer from seizures, do not use this species. If you must, only take the dosage amount that is in normal food.

Certain sage species contain Thujone. This chemical can trigger menstruation in a pregnant woman, which can easily lead to miscarriage. Therefore, it is advisable for pregnant woman and breastfeeding mothers not to consume sage. However, they can still have it for external use, as long as it will not get into their system.

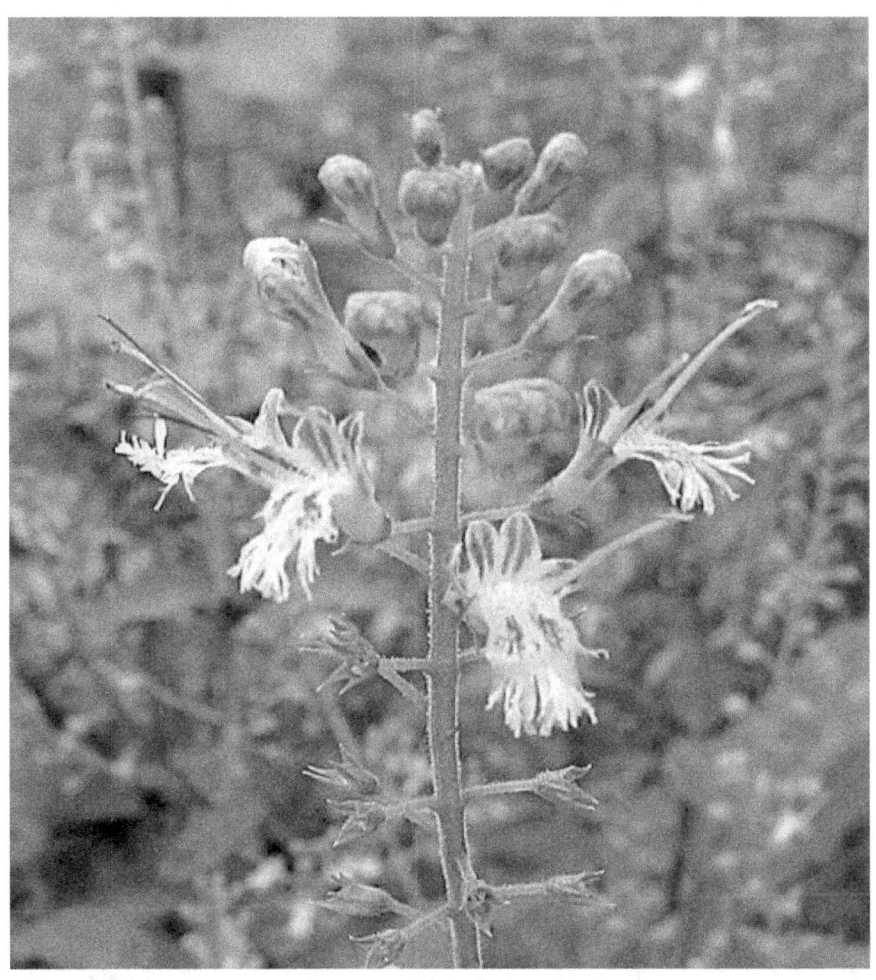

STONE ROOT

Also known as hardhack and richweed is another magnificent herb that has so much potential for curing certain aliments. The rootstock and leaves when extracted and processed can produce very tangible quantities of materials that has diuretic and astringent effects. Stone root is useful for taking care of problems that are kidney related. Most importantly, the herb is has a very strong effect on the mucous membrane and the nervous system. It is also very effective in the removal of congestions, and clearing the capillaries in order to improve the flow of blood in the body. This makes it one of the best remedies for health conditions like sore throat. You can also use it for gastritis and atonic dyspepsia.

Usage

People harvest Stone root herbs dried, which is very important so that the odor from the dried version will not be there again. Taking stone root for sore throat or any other ailments is good, as long as it is not an overdose.

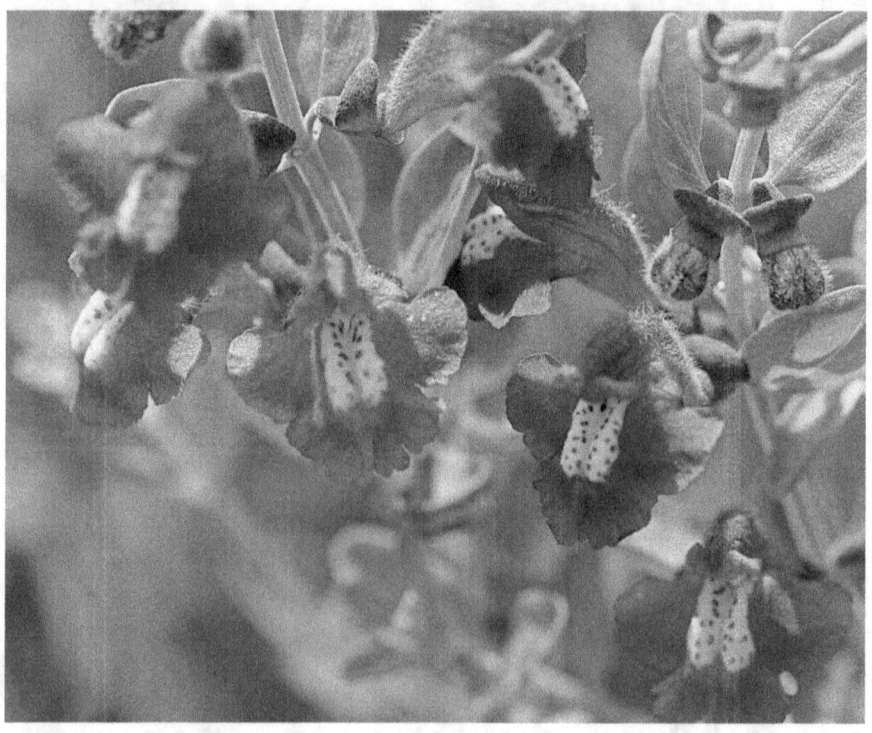

SKULLCAP

This herb is a mint, with very strong impact on some of the ailment we have today. The leaves, which come in different colors including blue, white and purple are the main parts used in the herb.

Skullcap anxiety and stress

The Native Americans know exactly what it means to be bundled with stress and anxiety, and the negative impact that it could have on the overall health and physical performance of the human being. Skullcap is very useful to relief stress and anxiety on the human body.

Cure for headaches and insomnia

The busy life of modern day people has made them very much succumb to the pressures of headaches and insomnia. Most people have tried multiple orthodox medicines to cure this, but it seems not effective. The natives used Skullcap to conquer insomnia and it is still very much effective until this day.

How to use skullcap

Just like many other herbs that have been modernized, skullcap is mostly is commonly consumed in the form of tea or supplement. The tea is easy because of the hot water dissolving process that ensures that the active ingredients find their way into your system. Teas and supplements also ensure that you don't take excess of the herb, which could lead to side effects.

Precautions

Just like many other herbs, it is advisable to consult your doctor first before you start taking skullcap. This is more important for people who are on other types of medications. You don't want drug reactions that might land you in very serious health problems. Skullcap has properties that slows down the central nervous system. This is why it is not recommended for both pregnant and breastfeeding women. You should also not take the herb during or after surgery.

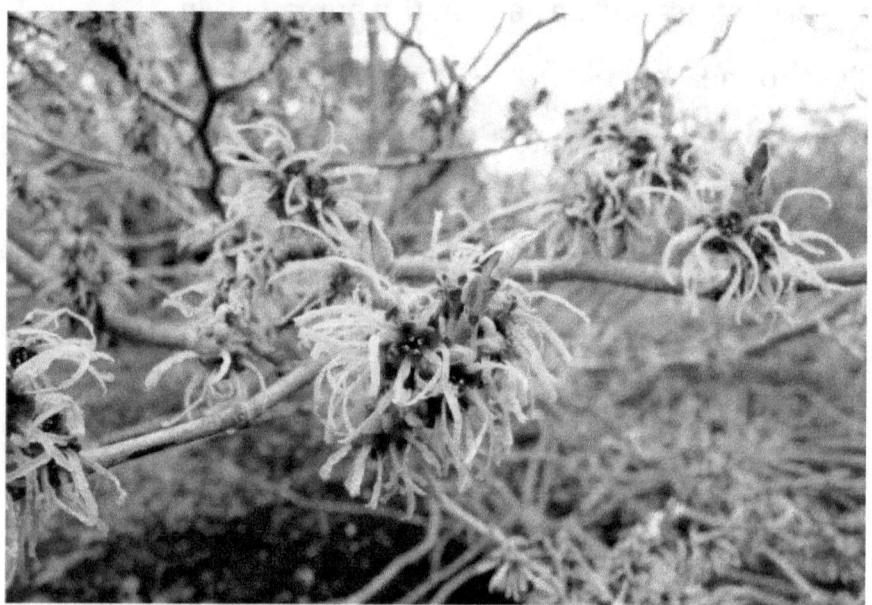

WITCH HAZEL

This is one of the herbs used by Native Americans for so many things. The twigs, bark and leaf are all harvested and then turn into medicine. Witch hazel is prepared for use after a proper extraction process. The active ingredient in the herb is a chemical known as Tannins, which is very effective in soothing skin infections, reducing swelling and getting rid of bacteria on the skin.

Five major uses of witch hazel

Many people are very familiar with Witch Hazel water, which is a made from the extracts derived from the bark and leaves of witch hazel. It makes a lot of sense to have any medicine made from witch hazel in your home, and here are five reasons why.

It works as a natural astringent

Your skin accommodates a lot of sweat and dust. When this mixes with the natural oil from the body, it can lead to skin infections. You can use Witch hazel on the skin to act as a natural astringent that can help eliminate excess oil. As you apply it on your skin, it will also help destroy the contaminant, so that you can reduce bacteria that enter your system through pores. Applying witch hazel on your skin can also prevent skin blemishes on the face e.g. blackheads.

Eye puffiness

Witch hazel has the ability to reduce or fight inflammation. This makes it very much suitable for taking care of discoloration and puffiness under the eye. You have to be careful when applying it, so that you don't get the substance into your eyes. This can lead to dryness and long-term pain.

Swollen veins

Are you suffering from varicose vein, just soak soft cloth into witch hazel and place it on the affected part, and see how you get fast relief.

Stop bleeding

People get cuts every day, from the kitchen to the garden. The faster you stop the bleeding, the better it is for your health. This is why it is very essential to have witch hazel in the house. All you have to do is apply it on the bleeding or minor cuts and experience faster healing. Organic witch hazel contains isopropyl alcohol. The alcohol makes it suitable for treating wounds and cut before applying bandage.

Damaged gums

Eating sweets, smoking and other poor eating habits can lead to serious gum problems. You can get rid of damaged gums with a moderate witch hazel mouthwash. This will help relieve the pain in your tooth and eliminate infections and irritations in and around your gums.

Other uses and precautions

Witch hazel is also effective for curing diaper's rash, sore throat, hemorrhoids relief, post hair-removal and treat bug bites and stings. Breastfeeding or pregnant women should not apply witch hazel for internal use. Adults and children can safely use it for external purposes. However, some people might experience skin rash due to excessive use.

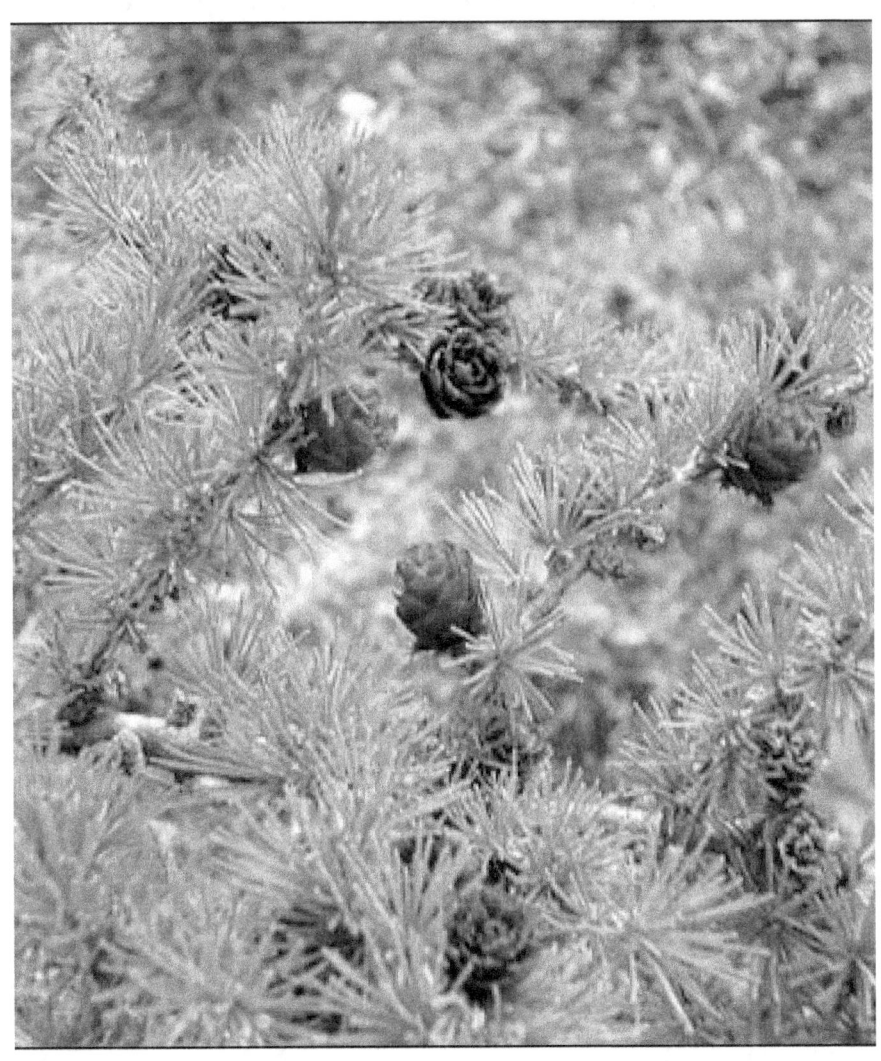

TAMARACK

This is one of the most useful herbs used in the past and in modern days. It grows in swampy areas and in slop areas too. In the old days, Native American from different tribes used this herb for a wide range of problems. You can use Tamarack tea, which has been made from extraction. The extracted substance is reputed to have a tonic, laxative and diuretic effect. The young shoot was used as emergency food for the locals, but the medicinal part is derived from the roots, bark and needle.

Common uses of Tamarack

Tamarac has been a subject of serious scientific research in recent years. The aim of this is to be able to find out why exactly the Native American tribes hold it so much in high esteem. Tamarack has proven to be very effective as it used to be, with the secrets of its powers becoming more and more available years after years.

Tamarack may help in the fight against cancer

Recent medical results show that tamarack may be very helpful in the fight against cancer. These claims have not been confirmed, but many medical practitioners and researchers who have taken part in experiments that have shown that tamarack is very promising when it comes to fighting cancer. The active ingredient that makes this possible is curcumin. This material helps to revitalize cells that can help fight cancer cells, a very important aspect of curing the diseases by boosting your immunity.

Dyspepsia

This term is used to generalize problems that are associated with digestive issues including bloating, gas and loss of appetite. Research shows that after taking about 500mg of tamarack on a daily basis, people who have bowel and digestive problems get sound relief within a period of one week. Sometimes, even a completely full relief is achieved.

Prevention of liver damage

The liver is a very important part of the human body, the most of which involves the removal of excess toxic waste. Research shows that people taking tamarack for a particular period may prevent their liver from damage. When this happens, people have to take caution. Because prolonged consumption of tamarack may lead to liver problems that can be very detrimental to the body. This is why, when taking tamarack for any problems, it is vital that you consult your doctor for advice on administration and prescriptions.

Parkinson's disease

Tamarack is helpful against Parkinson's disease. Researchers have found that the initial stages of Parkinson's involve the clumping of a certain protein. This clumping can be stopped by consuming certain amount of curcumins, which is abundantly available in the tamarack herb.

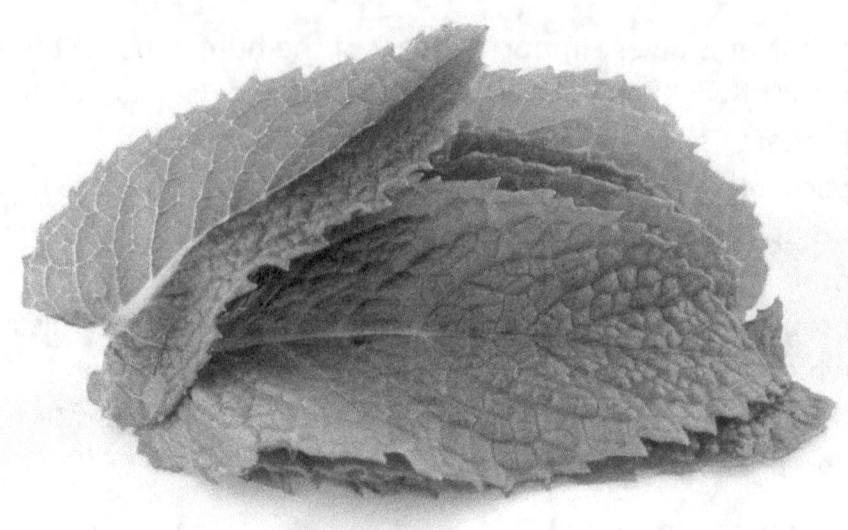

SPEARMINT

This herb is very popular for its leaves and oil, which is used as medicine. For thousands of years, generations of people have used it for a wide range of health issues. Spearmint derives its powers from the small amount of essential oils like Rosmarinic Acid and Carvone, which makes about 50% of its constituents.

Spearmint can be made into a nice herbal tea for internal consumption. It can also be included in baths, whether hot or cold.

What spearmint is used for?

Relieves indigestion

Indigestion troubles a whole lot of people in modern times. Why? Because people don't longer have the time to consume homemade natural foods anymore. Junks, fast food meals and other foods are one of the major causes of poor digestion in most people. The herb is very useful in curing digestive problems including gas, flatulence and loss of appetite. It can also help get rid of gall bladder inflammation, irritable bowel syndrome, nausea and indigestions.

Skin problems

Spearmint can be applied on the skin to help get rid of arthritis, muscle pains, nervous pains, swelling in the mouth and skin conditions like Urticaria.

Other uses

People use spearmint herb to cure toothache, sore throat, cramps, headache and inflammation of the respiratory tracts. Sometimes it can be tough getting rid of bad breathe with over-the-counter medicine. Spearmint can help you get rid of bad breath and save you from public embarrassment.

Precautions

If you have any kidney or liver disorders, it is very important that you seek the advice of your doctor before using spearmint. This is because excessive use of spearmint might increase kidney or liver problems and expose you to more dangers. You should also avoid using too much spearmint during pregnancy, as it can cause serious damage to your uterus.

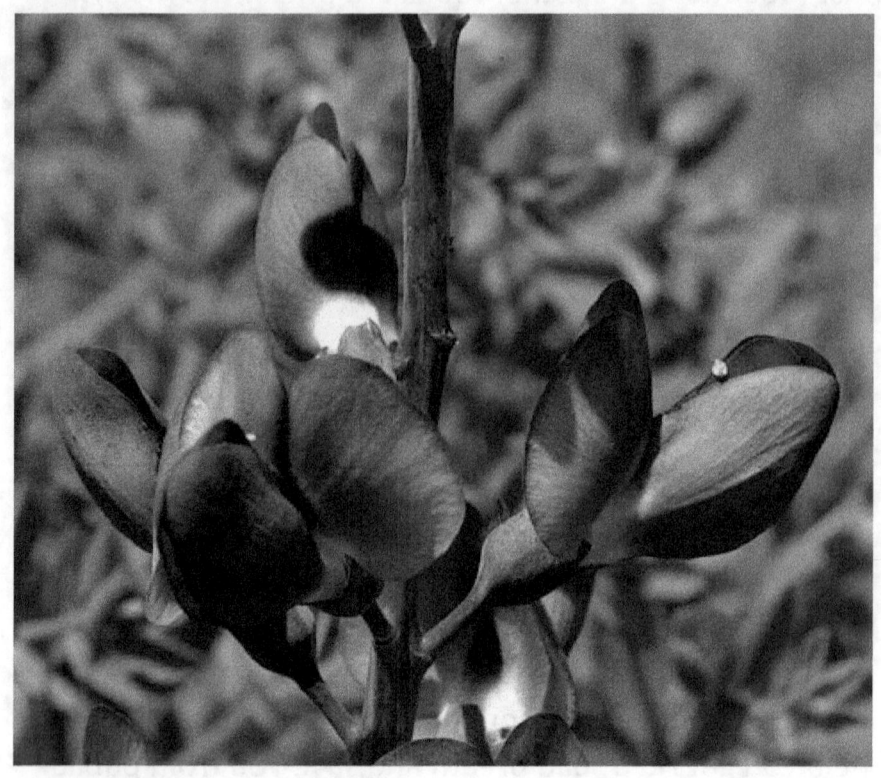

WILD INDIGO

The Native Americans used wild indigo roots as medicine for so many health issues. Wild indigo or American indigo, as it is sometimes called, is very effective against for certain purposes. It can be very effective for battling infectious diseases like swine flu, common flu, influenza, and many upper respiratory tract infections. It is also effective in the cure of typhoid fever, malaria, and scarlet fever and lymph node infections. It is also useful in treating throat infections, boils Crohn's disease and swelling in the mouth.

Some people also use wild indigo herbs on their skin to get rid of vaginal discharge, sores, painful nipples and ulcers. Sometimes wound can prove to be very difficult to heal, especially if you have a very soft skin surface. Using herbs like wild indigo has been shown to be very effective in the treatment and cleaning of open and swollen wounds.

Precautions

Just like many herbs, wild indigo is not good for breast feeding and nursing women, either internally or externally. People who have serious intestinal or stomach problems should also avoid taking the herb.

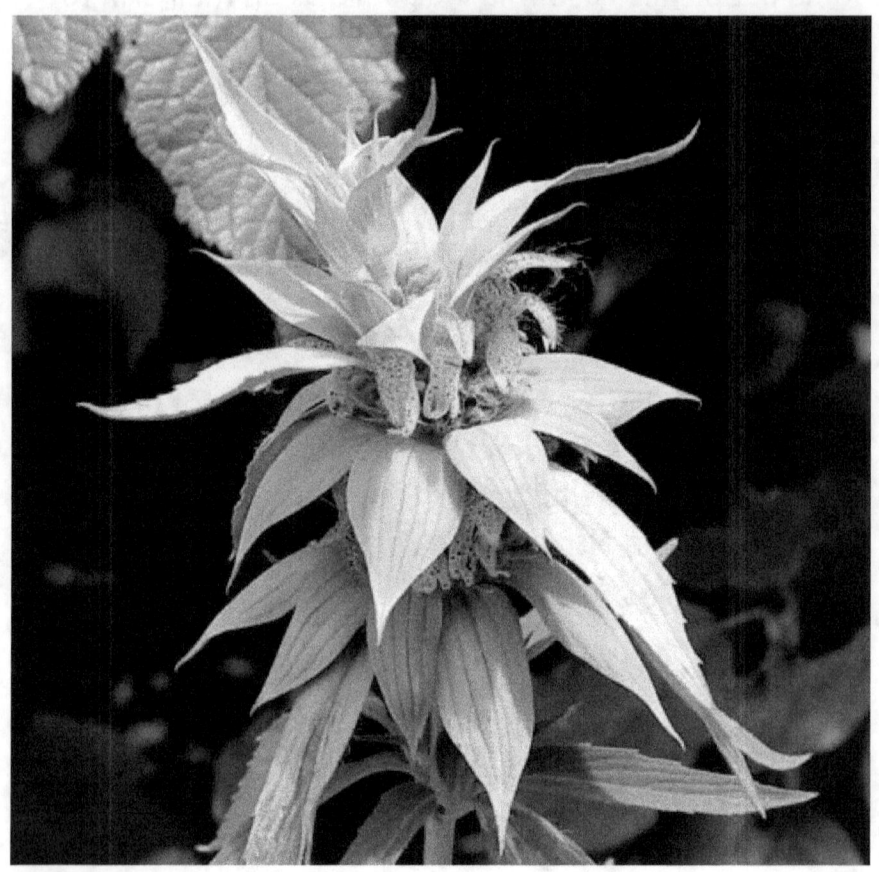

HORSEMINT

This herb from its name shows that it belongs to the mint family. Apart from being a useful ingredient in the kitchen, is has long been used for direct medicinal impact for many centuries.

Common uses of horsemint

Back pain

The Native Americans are very physically active so they suffer back pain issues. If you check medical statistics, you will find out that modern people are just about the same. Horsemint has soothing properties that make it excellent for curing back pains very fast, and with little effort.

Stomach cramp

Excessive cramps in the stomach can lead to serious problems that can be hard for sufferers to endure. When it becomes too common, it can be very annoying. Consuming horsemint as tea or supplement can help relief stomach cramps, and get to the root of the problem for a more permanent cure or solution.

Fever

The Native Americans suffer a lot from fever, so it makes sense that they have a long list of herbs they use to counter this disease. Consuming horsemint as tea, on a regular basis, can both prevent fever and help subside it. Horsemint is also known to cause sweating, which is believed to help remove the fever causing toxins in the body to guarantee healing.

Taking horsemint

Horsemint can be consumed as tea, supplement or extracts. The Native American chewed it, but that is not mostly common anymore. Now, people prefer to consume sweetened horsemint tea for better experience.

Precautions

Pregnant and breast feeding women should not take horsemint. Even though it is generally safe for consumption by adults, some people may experience stomach upset or nausea after taking horsemint.

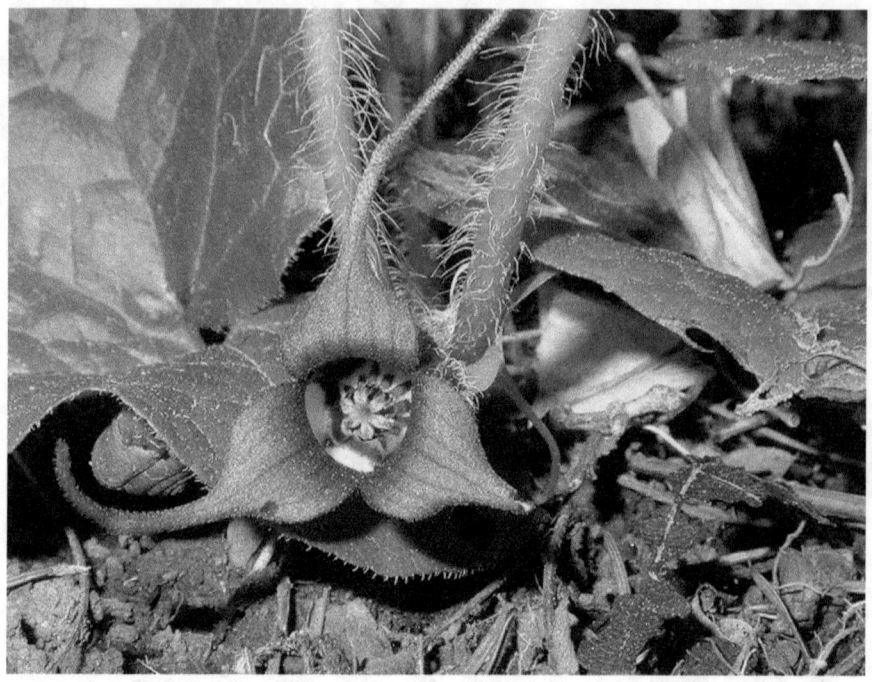

WILD GINGER

One of the reasons why Native American tribes have similar uses for so many herbs is because each tribe wanted to be different. After all, this is the only way to maintain your sovereignty and ensure that you are less dependent on almost everything. Wild ginger is one of the most widely used herbs by certain native tribes, and is still used up until this day. It is important to note that wild ginger got its name because the rhizome smells and tastes similar to that of ginger roots. Both plants are not related by any means.

Medical uses

The ancients prepared the roots of wild ginger rhizome to help bring relief to painful menstrual problems. It is also used to balance irregular heartbeats so that sufferers can live a more active life. They also made very effective tooth problem solutions by mixing wild ginger with other herbs derived from the bark of black alder, bayberry and black oak.

Candied wild ginger rhizome or syrup is used to cure stomach cramp and flatulence. According to "doctrines of signature" the kidney shape of the wild ginger must have influenced it been used to treat certain problems related to the kidney. Old Native American folklore also suggests that the wild ginger was used as an herb in the very common sweat lodge therapy, which involves getting rid of body toxins through sweating. It is also said to be effective in curing certain fevers and snakebites. Wild ginger is however most popular in modern times for the treatment of external health issues including gout and wounds.

Precautions

It is advisable that you seek medical consultation before using wild ginger. This is because it contains Aristolochic Acid, a naturally occurring toxin that can cause cancers and mutations in human cells.

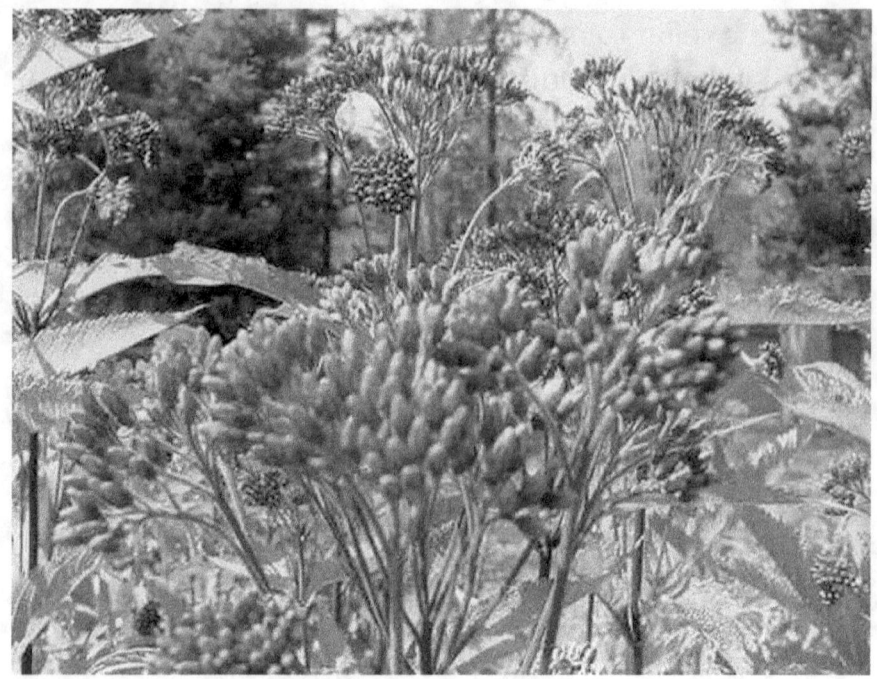

ASPEN

Aspen is a tree. The leaf and bark are medicinal, so it is cultivated to make herbs and very helpful medicine. Aspen contains a chemical known as Salicin. This Salicin is very much similar to aspirin, making it very helpful in the treatment of many cases of inflammation.

Uses of aspen

Pains

The Native Americans are very active people so they suffered a lot of pain, including joint pains and nerve pains. Aspen is known to be very effective in the cure of joint pains in most parts of the body. This is due to its high level of Salicin and other anti-inflammatory components that are abundant in the plant.

Nerve pains can be very uncomfortable. The Native Americans didn't have the proper technological devices and machinery to easily detect and find a cure for nerve pains. However, they still have a savior in aspen that help them get rid of the problem. If you're taking aspen for the first time, you'll find out that you'll be noticing relieve within half an hour. After your first and second dose, you will be getting results even faster than that.

Fever

Just like pains, the natives also suffered a lot in the hands of fever. The anti-inflammatory substances in aspen makes it easier to conquer fever and give relief within a very short time. This is much better than taking pills and drugs that are made from chemicals and will leave a negative effect on your body.

Other uses

Aspen is also indicated for curing bladder problems, nervous pain, prostrate discomfort and back troubles.

Precautions

It is advisable not to consume alcohol when using aspen. This is because the herb reacts with the stomach and intestine walls, thereby increasing the chances of internal bleeding. If you have any type of medical issues where aspirin usage is discouraged, you may also need to avoid aspen also. This is because of the Salicin in aspen, which is very similar in characteristics to aspirin. People with kidney problems, diabetes, gout, liver diseases, and stomach ulcers should not use aspen.

People with blood problems like hemophilia should avoid taking aspen because it can definitely make this type of blood disorder worse. If you have aspirin allergies, it is advisable that you also avoid taking aspen. Pregnant women and those who are breastfeeding advised to avoid consuming aspen for any reasons.

Taking aspen

There are several ways people administer aspen. The most common way is by applying a few drops on your few drops on pulse a major pulse point in your body e.g. the temple of your head. If you're taking it for internal use, you can do so by putting two drops under your tongue for maximum effects. People also take aspen by adding two drops into a small glass of water and sipping in little by little.

Aspen tea is also very common, and you can also purchase aspen supplement on the internet. Make sure that they are made from pure aspen herbs with little or no preservatives included.

CHAPTER 3

DETOX HEALING METHODS WITH SWEAT LODGE AND SAUNA

The Native Americans believe that in order to get cured, the human body must be made to align with nature or the spirits. They also believed that herbs have spirits, and that processing it the wrong way can make it lose its good spirit. These healing rituals involve the use of herbs, which are regarded as important to the specific ailment they are trying to cure.

SWEATING OUT IMPURITIES WITH THE SWEAT LODGE

When the European settlers arrived in native America, they bought with them so many things e.g. alcohol, which is considered as impure by most Native American tribes. They felt that being exposed to such things made them impure, so, they need to find a way to get rid of the impurities before it drags them away from the ways of the spirits and ancestors. Taking part in the sweat lodge will help you sweat out toxins, to attain a better physical and mental health.

The sweat lodge is a small hut built from thick parts of herbs, and made to contain a number of people. The hut is filled with heated stones, which releases heat, so that the people in it can become hot and then release sweat. While inside the hut, participants are expected to say prayers, asking for new guidance from the spirits, to provide answers that can lead to complete purification. At the end, people leaving the hut feel refreshed and energized to continue in the right ways of their ancestors.

After the sweat lodge is closed, people are advised to excuse themselves if they cannot handle it. All they need is to make a signal and the rest of the occupants will create a way for them to exit.

SAUNAS ARE THE MODERN SWEAT LODGE

In modern time, it is difficult to access a real sweat lodge. Most people have to travel far distances where Native American medicine men and women still exist, before they can find one. However, you can still make use of a sauna in order to achieve a similar purpose.

The sauna works on the same principle as the sweat lodge. Heat is generated so that the skin can produce enough sweat, thereby eliminating toxins along with it. So how does this work?

The skin is the largest organ in the body. One of its main functions is to help eliminate excess water, along with unwanted substances from the body. The kidney, liver, lungs and bowels also share in this responsibility. Sweating is also important for the body because the skin uses it to cool our temperature so as not to put vital organs in danger. The skin also has the ability to transform toxins that are oil-based into water-soluble forms that can easily be eliminated by the body.

WHAT ARE THE BENEFITS OF SAUNA BATHS?

Natural healing

Perhaps, one of the most dangerous behavior of modern people is the relentless desire to find the shortest route to a healthy solution. People in years past have relied mainly on nature for their healing, and it had benefited them very much. This is evident in the long years of living, which is a rare thing for modern people.

Sauna baths is the body safe and natural way to heal itself. This happens when the body eliminates all the toxins in it, so that the cells begin to work at a higher frequency. Scientists are beginning to realize how beneficial sweating can be, when it comes to getting rid of toxins. This is perhaps one of the reasons why physical exercises work, as it involves a lot of sweating.

Remove toxins

Our modern world is filled with chemicals, which are part of our food, liquids, shampoo, soap, body wash and body lotion and cream. These chemicals find their way into our body through the pores in our skin, and then become toxic and become a threat to our healthy living.

Taking part in sauna baths can help you eliminate such toxins with little or no effort. Remember, some of these toxins may not be detectable when we go for tests or something, but are actually contributing to our ill health in no small amount. Sometimes, the orthodox drugs we use, after doing their work, leave some remnants in our body, which actually become toxins. A sauna bath can help eliminate these toxins and set you on a greater path to good health.

Improved blood circulation

Surely, exposing your body to heat will melt down fats that have accumulated in different parts of your body. The major among them are the fat that have deposited on the linings of your blood vessel so that proper blood circulation is hindered. The melting down of this fat will ensure a widening of the blood vessel so that blood can flow very easily. Improved blood circulation will definitely lead to better immunity, more energy and increased cellular activities.

Weight loss

There is a huge similarity between sauna and mild exercise. Being that you're generating heat to melt down fat. Experts have found out that a single session of sauna can help you lose at least 300 calories. If you now combine that with physical exercise and a healthy diet, you can be guaranteed of quick weight loss that will help ensure a healthy lifestyle.

Skin cleansing

Showers are good, but what about taking a shower after a sauna session. The sauna bath ensures that you have a much cleaner skin that will provide better protection against chemical creeping into your body. Your skin will also become more fresh and attractive, so that you will rely less on artificial in order to make your beauty visible.

Body and mind relaxation

Modern life has taken a toll on the human race. This leads to stress, which also leads to other more dangerous diseases that leads to death. Stress that is in the form of tension is hard to deal with, even with orthodox medicine. This is because it involves more of the inner part of a human being, which is not very easy to access.

Sauna bath can be very helpful in relieving the symptoms of stress and causes, which may include pain in the body, tense muscle and sore limbs. The heat and humidity of the sauna have the ability to penetrate into different parts of the body, so it can help you attain higher relaxation and ease. The sauna is a quiet place, so it provides the perfect space for relaxation. People who regularly make use of saunas agree that it is the perfect place to get complete relief from mental and physical fatigue and stress.

CHAPTER 4

YOUR JOUNEY TO A COMPLETELY HEALTHY LIFE

KNOW BEFORE YOU TAKE A DECISION

For the many people that try out Native medicines without success, it is mostly because of the lack of knowledge. People are very much emotional about things, jumping into conclusions and following the crowd, just because of some testimonial.

Native American medicines have been used for years. Even though its effects may not be as serious as it were thousands of years ago, due to poor data keeping, but people have testified to its potency. Then, you can't just jump on the bandwagon. You need to get yourself educated first before taking any native medicine.

Get a diagnosis

The first thing you want to do is to find out about your disease. You want to do as many tests as required, so that you'll know exactly what is wrong or right with you. You want to know everything as much as you can. This is why you have to work very closely with your doctor, so that there will be some monitoring as you embark on this journey into healing by nature. Once you understand what you're dealing with, you can now move into the next stage.

Understand your ailment and healing options

Most people that seek native medicine have it in mind that because it is nature, it is far better than orthodox medicine. While this may be true for some medical issues, it may not be true for all. For example, there are situations or health problems that will certainly require a medical surgery before it will go. There are no alternatives. If you are in this type of situation, it will do you good to consider surgery first.

Understanding your ailment also ensures that errors are limited or cut down to zero. No matter how determined you think you are, the nature of your ailment will always be the major determinant to know if it is something you should wholly subject to treatment through herbs.

Do research

In addition to working with your doctor, you should also try do your own research about what is wrong with you. This is even more important for people who have been dealing with certain ailments for a very long time. Your research should be on the causes, triggers, and prevention options of your ailment. If your doctor thinks that you should try conventional medicine first, you can go on with it as long as you can afford it. If not, you still need to discuss with your doctor about herbals - and how you are going to use it the right way.

WHO SHOULD CONSIDER NATIVE AMERICAN MEDICINE?

There are certain groups of people who should consider Native American medicines more. Of course, it is available for all, but these people should take it even more seriously as it could be the very lasting solution to their problems.

You've tried conventional medicine without changes.

Evidence has shown that some people suffering from seemingly minor ailments had struggled with it for years, without any proper results. For example, many people have reported dealing with insomnia, migraine or headaches for years, without finding a solution after taking plenty of pills. If you fall into this category, it is important that you consider alternative medicine like the Native American medicine. You need to discuss with your doctor about options before moving on to the alternative way.

You're tired of taking pills

Some people have taken pills so much that it has become a mental burden. Yes, if you find solid information about natural remedies, it is normal to feel that you want to get rid of the chemicals. Native medicine offers you the opportunity to try out nature, in its unprocessed form. Our body contains similar elements that are available in nature. This makes it safe and acceptable by our internal organs.

You hate drug side effects

Many conventional medicines have side effects that might even be worse than the ailment itself. Some people have endured sleepless nights, skin rash, stomach upset, headaches, nausea, vomiting, itching etc. just because they want to get a cure. Most herbs don't have serious side effects, unless you didn't take them in moderations. In fact, there are herbs that can help you overcome some of the side effects caused by the use of conventional medicine.

You want a combination

Sometimes your prescriptions may be working perfectly, but you still want to include natural herbs. You need to talk to your doctor and see how this works out. Self-medication in any form is dangerous. Not to talk of herbs that you have no idea what they contain. Your doctor will be able to guide you in the kind of herbs you can take. He will also guide you on how to make it work with your pills. Many people have experienced faster recovery, less drug side effects and better drug assimilation when they did it right.

You want to save money

Conventional medicine is expensive. Perhaps, this is among the reasons why many people want to try out alternative medicines, which can provide the same results with a smaller bill. Understandably, alternative medicine is cheaper because it is made from nature. The raw materials are derived from plants, trees, leaves and roots that cost little to nothing to get.

The manufacturing and process is also very easy, and most times the herbs come with their own natural preservatives, so that they don't get spoilt for a very long time. Alternative medicine can save you a lot of money and at the same time give you even more relief compared to what conventional medicine can do for you.

You want to try out new things

If you have been using pills all your life for minor aliment like headaches, pain, sore throat, and cold, it is a great thing for anyone to try out. You'll be doing some exciting experiment with your body, and will be able to measure the difference between both methods. Trying out alternative medicine will also help you discover new things about your body. The more new things you discover about yourself, the healthier you'll live. No doubt about that.

IMPORTANT THINGS TO REMEMBER WHEN TAKING NATIVE AMERICAN MEDICINE

Just like your conventional medicine, native medicine also requires some special attentions and considerations, if you really want it to work. These are the points you must put at the back of your mind to help you harness the power of herbs.

Consult your doctor

Never take any herb until you consult your doctor; this fact can never be overemphasized. Don't be fooled by the idea that we are part of nature, so, it is safe no matter how you do it. No, it is not. Even if it does, you never can know if you have an ailment that cannot withstand the ingredients of the herb, thereby making your condition worse.

Herbs have side effects too

Yes, they do. Some herbs contain very powerful chemicals in natural form, which can cause serious harm if consumed in a large quantity. In fact, most herbs are medicinal when consumed in small quantities, but dangerous if consumed in large quantities. To avoid side effects, make sure you equip yourself with the right knowledge about your body, the herb and your ailment before you start taking them. You should also discuss with your doctor so you can get the perfect dosage requirements for yourself.

What worked for others may not work for you

Don't say because you read about a testimonial online, or you saw a video about someone benefiting from an herb and you want to do the same. What worked for someone may not necessarily work for you. This is because we humans have different body chemistry, and we react to medication very differently. Find what works for you and stick to it. Including sticking to the method of application that best works for you.

HARVESTING AND STORING YOUR HERBS

Medicinal herbs like Native American medicines require very delicate handling when harvesting and storing them. This is to ensure that they do not lose their active properties and then become useless or ineffective when you really need them. You want to ensure that you harvest and then store them properly. Some people prefer to just buy them in the market and use them. Alternatively, you can just buy the dried ones that are in the form of tea. If that is what you want to do, fine. However, if you really want to have a complete advantage of the herbs by planting them then, you'll need to know how to carry out the process the right way.

Harvesting

Herbs are most useful for medicinal purpose when dried. But then, you still need to harvest them the right way. Avoid harvesting your herbs when they are still wet because they can easily mildew. You should also not wait until the sun is high before harvesting. Also, do not harvest them just before blooming. This is because the period signified they are trying to reproduce and would have invested all their energy and nutrients in the process.

Best time to harvest herbs is in the morning just after the sun sets out. The sun would have dried them just enough to be ready for harvesting.

Drying

You can easily dry herbs with low moisture content by laying them in the open air. Herbs with higher moisture content, like the ones with roots, will require a dehydrator if you want them to dry properly.

Before drying your herbs, make sure that you remove the bad parts like leaves and roots. Store them under a temperature of 90 to 100 degrees Fahrenheit. You must ensure that there is proper air circulation, at your preferred drying spot, to guarantee that the herbs dry well.

Storing

Once your herbs are dried and ready to preserve, you can store them in airtight Ziploc bags and canning jars. It is important that you select jars that are rigid, to prevent crushing or damaging of the herbs. Make sure that you label all herbs before storing them. It is advisable that you do not grind your herb or turn them into powder form, until you are ready to consume them. Most of the storage instructions can also be very helpful for people who will be buying the dried herbs and storing them for future use.

CONCLUSION

Native American medicine is an opportunity for people to discover new ways to tackle their ailments and find a natural solution to their health challenges. Many herbs can be used to tackle this. Before you make a move, it is important that you considered getting some knowledge first. Know what it is exactly that you're suffering from. Discuss with your doctor about options and choose what will best work for you. Always ensure that whatever you consume is the right proportion.

If you have gone through conventional means without any positive result, then you should try out Native American medicines. Many ailments that we have today were treated long ago. It is just that the process of application may have been lost, due to many factors that includes disrupting the natural lifestyle of the Native American tribes.

If you have any question, you should direct them to your medical doctor. He will be able to guide you through every inch of the process and help you find the perfect herb to provide exactly that type of healing that you're looking for. In addition to taking herbs, you should also not neglect other very beneficial health activities like exercise, good diet and proper sleep and rest. This will not only facilitate your healing, but will ensure that it lasts for a very long time.

Live a healthy and fulfilling lifestyle. Be happy and smile a lot. If you feel stressed out, take a deep breath or go stay alone by the sea. Remember, herbs work with nature.

Therefore, as you consume them, they rely on your connection with nature to be able to work effectively. Give yourself some time to heal and don't ever rush herbs. You can achieve the ultimate health desire that you want as long as you follow the right instructions, listen to your doctor and pay attention to your body.

www.ingramcontent.com/pod-product-compliance
Lightning Source LLC
Chambersburg PA
CBHW071142280526
45787CB00003B/1371